HEALTHY CROCK POT

RECIPES 2021

FLAVORFUL RECIPES FOR YOUR CROCK POT

BOB MALONE

Chicken Mole

Source: Everyday Foods

Ingredients

- 4 pounds organic chicken thighs, boneless, skinless

- sea salt

- 1 can (28 oz) whole tomatoes

- 1 medium yellow onion, roughly chopped

- 2 dried ancho chiles, stemmeds

- 1 large chipotle chile in adobo sauce

- 1/2 cup sliced almonds, toasted

- 1/4 cup raisins

- 3 ozs bittersweet or dark chocolate (dairy- and soy-free), chopped

- 3 garlic cloves, peeled and smasheds

- 3 Tbs extra virgin olive oil

- 3/4 tsp cumin

-

1/2 tsp cinnamon

-

fresh cilantro, for serving optional

Preparation

1.

Season chicken with salt and place in a 5-6 quart slow cooker.

2.

In a blender, puree all remaining ingredients, except cilantro until smooth. Add tomato mixture to the slow cooker, cover, and cook on high until chicken is tender, about 4 hours on high (8 hours on low).

3.

Serve with rice and topped with cilantro.

Honey Glazed Chicken Thighs

Ingredients

1 teaspoon Kosher Salt

1 teaspoon Black Pepper

1 teaspoon Red Pepper Flakes

1 teaspoon Chili Powder

2 teaspoons Paprika

2 teaspoons Garlic Powder

½ cups Honey

2 tablespoons Apple Cider Vinegar

3 pounds Chicken, Thighs, Boneless/Skinless

Freezer Containers

2 Gallon Freezer Bags

Preparation

1.
Mix salt, pepper, red pepper flakes, chili powder, paprika and garlic powder together and set aside. Mix honey and cider vinegar and set aside. Un-tuck chicken thighs so they are flat.

2.
Cover both sides in seasoning and place chicken in slow cooker. Pour honey mixture over chicken.

3.

Cook on low for 6-8 hours or on high for 3-4 hours. If you are able to baste the chicken by spooning some of the liquid over the chicken periodically during the cooking time, please do.

4.

Take chicken out of slow cooker and let rest for a few minutes.

5.

Spoon excess glaze over chicken before serving.

Mini Turkey Meatballs

Ingredients

- pound 99% lean ground turkey breast

- pound 94% lean ground turkey

- 2/3 cup cooked quinoa (preferably cooked in flavored stock)

- garlic cloves, minced or pressed

- large egg, lightly beaten

- tablespoons olive oil

- tablespoons finely grated romano cheese

- teaspoons dried basil

- teaspoon dried oregano

- 1/2 teaspoon onion powder

- 1/2 teaspoon salt

-

1/2 teaspoon pepper

-

large sweet onion, sliced into thin rounds

-

(28 ounce) cans crushed tomatoes

Preparation

1.

In a large bowl, combine turkey, quinoa, garlic, beaten egg, olive oil, cheese, basil, oregano, salt and pepper.

2.

Mix thoroughly but quickly, just so the ingredients are combined - do not overmix! Roll into mini balls - slightly smaller than a golfball, and place on a baking sheet.

3.

Layer sliced onion on the bottom of the crockpot and add 1 can of crushed tomatoes.

4.

Heat a large skillet over medium-high heat and add 1/2 tablespoon olive oil.

5.

Add meatballs, searing on the top and bottom until golden, about 1 minute per side.

6.

To flip meatballs, gently toss with a spoon.

7.

Add meatballs one at a time to the crockpot. Repeat with remaining meatballs - it is okay to stack them once they are all finished.

8.

Once all the meatballs are in the crockpot, add the other can of crushed tomatoes, completely submerging the meatballs. Cook on low for 6 hours.

Parmesan Chicken

Ingredients

- 4 boneless, skinless chicken breasts

- 4 tablespoons olive oil

- 6 tablespoons dry white wine

- 1/2 teaspoon salt

- 1/2 teaspoon pepper

- 4 garlic cloves, minced

- teaspoon dried basil

- 1/2 teaspoon dried parsley

- 1/4 cup finely grated parmesan cheese + 2 tablespoons

- cup uncooked whole wheat orzo

- 3/4 cup vegetables of your choice

Preparation

1.

The night before, season chicken breasts with salt and pepper.

2.

Whisk together 3 tablespoons olive oil, cheese, basil, parsley, garlic and 3 tablespoons of wine in a bowl.

3.

Place chicken in a large ziplock bag, then pour marinade over top and coat chicken. Keep in the fridge overnight.

4.

The next morning, place chicken in your crockpot with 3 tablespoons of wine.

5.

Cook on low for 6-8 hours.

6.

Prepare whole wheat orzo according to directions. Once cooked, combine with remaining olive oil, parmesan and salt and pepper if desired.

7.

Cut chicken into pieces/chunks, and toss together with orzo.

Chicken Cordon Bleu

Ingredients

☐

4-6 Boneless, skinless Chicken Breasts

☐

4 to 6 slices Swiss or Provolone cheese

☐

4 to 6 thin slices smoked ham

☐

1/4 to 1/2 cup all-purpose flour to coat the chicken

Sauce

☐

1 Cup milk

☐

1 cup heavy cream

☐

1 cup chicken broth

☐

1 1/2 cups Cheddar, Swiss or Colby cheese-grated (I used swiss slices)

☐

1/2 cup of grated Parmesan cheese (opt)

☐

2-4 tablespoons butter

☐

2 heaping tablespoons flour

☐

1 tsp. sauteed onions or minced onions

⁇
1/2 tsp. pepper

⁇
1 tsp. salt

⁇
2 teaspoons white granulated sugar

Instructions:

1.

Place chicken breasts between sheets of plastic wrap. Using a mallet, pound each chicken breast to 1/4" thickness.

2.

Place 1 cheese slice and 1 ham slice on each breast. Roll up each breast and using a toothpick, secure the ends, then coat each in roll of chicken in flour & shake off any excess.

3.

In a large skillet, add a few tablespoons of butter and turn your heat to med/high.

4.

When the butter is melted and hot, carefully place your chicken rolls in the skillet and brown both sides of the chicken.

5.

Once they are a nice golden color, add chicken to crock pot. Make sure you remember to remove the toothpicks!

Sauce:

1.

In a saucepan over medium/high heat, melt butter and add the salt, pepper, onions and the sugar and whisk to combine.

2.

Add the flour, and whisk quickly until bubbly and smooth.

3.

Add the broth, cream & milk and keep on whisking over med. heat until it has thickened.

4.

Add grated cheese (or cheese slices) and stir until melted and sauce is smooth and creamy.

5.

Pour the sauce over chicken and cover.

6.

Cook on low for 5-6 hours or on high for 3-4 hours.

Easy Pepper Steak

- lb. Beef, Round Steak, lean

- 3/4 c. bell pepper, green, strips

- 1/2 c. bell pepper, red, strips

- 1/2 c. bell pepper, yellow, strips

- 1/2 c. onion, sliced

- clove garlic

- 6 T. soy sauce

- T. pepper, black

Preparation

1.

Cut round steak, peppers and onions into strips.

2.

Sear steak in pan over med. high heat (optional).

3.

Press clove of garlic into crock, add all ingredients.

4.

Cover. Cook on Low for 8-10 hours.

Mongolian Beef

Ingredients

- 1/2 lb. steak, flank

- garlic cloves, minced

- 1/2 c. carrots, shredded

- onion, green, sliced, one is for garnish

- tsp. onion, dried minced (or 1/2 fresh onion, diced very small)

- 1/2 c. soy sauce, gluten free

- 1/4 c. wine, white

- 1/4 c. cooking sherry

- 1/2 T. vinegar, white wine(optional)

- tsp. sesame oil

- tsp. molasses

-

tsp. ginger

-

1/4 tsp. black pepper

-

tsp. red chili pepper flakes

-

1/2 T. peanut butter (if allergic, use black bean paste)

-

T. brown sugar

-

1/4 c. cornstarch (to dredge meat--don't add to sauce mixture)

Preparation

1.
Slice steak into thin strips and toss in a Ziploc bag with cornstarch to coat.

2.
Add all of the liquid and dried spices to your slow cooker, and the peanut butter (or alternative if necessary), and mix well.

3.
Add the garlic, carrots and three of the sliced green onions. If you are using fresh onion, add that at this time, too.

4.
Place the steak on top, and toss gingerly to coat.

5.
Cover. Cook on low for 4-6 hours.

Round Steak

- 1 ½ pounds round steak, cut into 3 inch chunks

- 1 medium onion chopped

- 3 cloves of garlic, minced

- 1 teaspoon dried thyme

- 1 teaspoon dried basil

- 2 cups beef broth

- ½ cup red wine

For last 30 minutes cooking

- ¼ cup cornstarch

- ¼ cup water

Preparation

1.

Place meat and onion in crockpot.

2.

Combine remaining ingredients, except water and cornstarch, and pour over meat and onion.

3.

Cook on low for 6-7 hours or until meat is tender. 30 minutes before serving, combine water and cornstarch and add to meat mixture.

4.

Cook on high for 30 minutes, this will thicken the sauce.

5.

Serve over rice, noodles, or grits.

Chipotle Beef Tacos

Ingredients

⬚
3 lbs ground beef

⬚
1 onion, finely chopped

⬚
8 ounces tomato sauce

⬚
2 chipotle peppers (this is 2 peppers not 2 cans)

⬚
1 teaspoon cumin

⬚
¾ teaspoon salt

Preparation

1.
Cook ground beef and onion in a skillet until the meat is no longer pink and the onion is tender. Set aside.

2.
In a food processor or blender puree tomato sauce, peppers, cumin, and salt.

3.

Combine pureed sauce and ground beef and place in a slow cooker. Cook on low for 3-4 hours.

4.

Serve with beans, lettuce, cheese, etc as tacos with tortilla shells or use with tostada shells.

5.

The leftover filling freezes really well.

Beef Fajitas

Ingredients

☐
2 ½ pound beef roast (I used rib roast, but any cut will do)

☐
4 ounces diced green chilies

☐
3 sweet peppers sliced

☐
1 yellow onion sliced

☐
3 tablespoons chili powder

☐
3 teaspoons cumin

☐
2 teaspoons salt

☐
2 teaspoons paprika

☐
1 teaspoon garlic powder

☐
1 teaspoon onion powder

☐
1 teaspoon pepper

☐
Squirt of lime juice

�

Tortillas

⁊

Fajita Fixings: sour cream, cheese, salsa, lettuce, etc.

Preparation

1.
Place the roast in the bottom of your crock. Place vegetables around the sides of the roast.

2.
In a small bowl, combine the chili powder through pepper. Stir well. Sprinkle over meat and veggies.

3.
Spoon chilies over top. Give it all a good squirt of lime juice. Cover and cook on low for 8 hours.

4.
Remove meat from crock. Shred with two forks. Drain juices from crock, leaving a small amount. Stir beef back in.

5.
Serve beef on tortillas with desired sides.

Simple Greek-Inspired Beef Roast

Ingredients:

▢

3 pounds beef roast

▢

1/3 cup olive oil, butter, or other fat (here's a frugal healthy fat!)

▢

3/4 cup onion, chopped

▢

6-7 whole cloves

▢

5-6 peppercorns

▢

1 two or three inch-long cinnamon stick (sounds unusual but trust me – it's good)

▢

1 ½ – 2 cups tomato juice (I've successfully substituted diced tomatoes)

▢

Salt and pepper, to taste

Directions:

1.

Pour half of the oil in the bottom of a large skillet and brown the roast on the skillet, using tongs to carefully flip it over and brown it on all sides.

2.

Place browned roast in the bottom of your slow cooker and add tomato juice, cloves, peppercorns, and cinnamon.

3.

Pour the rest of the oil into the skillet and sauté the onions until translucent.

4.

Pour the onions on top of the roast, scraping the sides of the skillet to get any extra oil or fat to add to the slow cooker.

5.

Cover and cook on low 6-8 hours. Add salt and pepper to taste and serve over brown rice (with a Simple Greek Salad, if desired).

Cajun Roast

Ingredients

- 1 roast of your choice (2 – 2 ½ pounds)

- 1 teaspoon cumin

- 1 teaspoon chili powder

- ½ teaspoon onion powder

- ½ teaspoon garlic powder

- ¼ teaspoon pepper

- ½ teaspoon salt

- 2 cups corn

- ½ cup chopped onion

- ½ cup chopped green pepper

- 1 tomato diced

◌
Rice to serve

Directions:

1.
Combine spices.

2.
Put roast in greased crock pot. Pour half of your spices over the roast. Rub in. Flip roast and coat with remaining spices, rubbing in well.

3.
Pour veggies (excluding corn) over the roast.

4.
Layer the corn over the top.

5.
Cover and cook on low for 8-10 hours or until temp reads 160+ degrees.

6.
Serve over a bed of rice.

Stuffed Peppers

- 4-5 medium sized peppers

- 1 ½ cups cooked black beans, rinsed

- 1 cup shredded cheese

- ¾ cup salsa

- ½ cup corn

- 1 cup cooked brown rice

- 1 teaspoon chili powder

- 1 teaspoon cumin

- ½ pound of cooked ground meat, if desired

- Sour cream, for serving (optional)

Directions:

1.

Wash and gut the peppers.

2.

In a large bowl, combine the rice, cheese, beans, salsa, corn, chili powder, and cumin (ground meat if desired). Stir.

3.

Stuff peppers with mixture.

4.

Place peppers in crock.

5.

Add ¼ cup of water to the bottom of the crock.

6.

Cover and cook on Low for 3-4 hours or until peppers are tender. Serve with sour cream if desired

Cube Steak

- 1 pkg (6-8 pc) cube steak

- 1 Onion, sliced

- 2 Cans Cream of Mushroom Soup (Stacy uses Homemade Cream of Mushroom Soup)

- 1 Cup Beef Broth

- 16 oz fresh mushrooms, sliced

- ½ cup flour

- ¼ tsp salt

- ½ tsp pepper

- 2 TBSP olive oil

- Sour Cream (optional)

- Cooked noodles

Directions:

1.

In a shallow dish or on a plate, combine the flour, salt and pepper. Heat the olive oil in a large skillet over medium-high heat.

2.

While it is heating, begin dredging the steaks in the flour, coating both sides well, and then place in the hot oil to brown. Turn once a nice crust has formed.

3.

While the steaks are browning, slice the onion.

4.

Next, layer half of the browned steaks, half of the onions, half of the mushrooms, and half of the cream of mushroom soup. And, you guessed it, repeat the layers.

5.

Turn the heat up just a tad, pour the broth (or whatever you are using) into the searing hot skillet and scrub the bottom of the pan with a wooden spoon to get it all up and mixed together well. When all the little bits are scraped up, pour the whole lot of it over the top of the ingredients in the crock-pot.

6.

You can cook it on high for 4-6 hours, or put it on low for 8-12 hours.

7.

This makes a lot of sauce, so I serve it over noodles. And I love this with sour cream; you could mix it in right before serving or just throw some on top of each serving.

GINGER BEEF

Makes: 3 entrees, 6 servings each.

Source: Fix, Freeze, Feast by Kati Neville and Lindsay Tkacsik

Ingredients

- 6 pounds sirloin tip beef or other beef suitable for slow cooking

- 3 cups water

- 9 scallions chopped (about 1 1/2 cups)

- 3/4 cup soy sauce

- 6 tsp beef bouillon granules

- 6 tsp minced ginger

- 6 tsp minced garlic

- 3 one-gallon freezer bags

Directions

1.
Rinse and trim beef as desired. Cut into thick strips, about 2×5 inches (The beef should not be in bite-size pieces.) Divide beef evenly among the 1-gallon freezer bags.

2.
Into each bag of beef measure 1 cup water, 1/2 cup scallions, 1/4 cup soy sauce, 2 tsp bouillon, 2 tsp ginger, and 2 tsp garlic.

3.
Seal and freeze.

Cooking

1.
Thaw one entree in the refrigerator, or cook it straight from the freezer.

2.
Put beef and broth into slow cooker. Cook on low for 5-6 hours, or until beef is fork tender.

Beef Enchiladas

Ingredients:

- 1 ½ lb ground beef

- 1 large onion, chopped

- 4 cloves garlic, minced

- 32 ounces homemade or all-natural enchilada sauce or salsa (we like tomatillo salsa!)

- 1 cup crème fraiche (or real sour cream: ingredients should say "cream, culture")

- 1 ½ cups refried beans (homemade, if possible!)

- 2-3 cups shredded cheddar (buy good quality and shred it yourself)

- One dozen homemade tortillas or all-natural from the store

Instructions:

1.
Brown the meat, drain and set aside.

2.
Saute the onions and garlic in butter until soft, then return the meat to the pan. Add the sauce or salsa and the crème fraiche. Simmer for 10 minutes.

3.
In a buttered crockpot, put a thin layer of sauce, then layer in this order: tortillas, refried beans, meat sauce and cheese. Repeat until all ingredients are used, ending with cheese.

4.
Cook on low 5 hours.

5.
Serve with fresh cilantro, more crème fraiche and lacto-fermented salsa.

Mexican Stew Meat

Ingredients

- 4+ onions

- 4-6 tomatillos

- 4+ peppers (any variety)

- Several Cloves of Garlic Crushed

- Salt

- Pepper

- Pounds Beef Stew Meat (or other meat of choice)

Directions:

1.

Blend all vegetables in a blender until pureed to your liking, (smooth, chunky or in between).

2.

Place the meat in the slow cooker, sprinkle with salt and pepper then pour the vegetable puree over all.

3.

Cover and cook on low for 6-8 hours.

4.

Serve in warm tortillas!

Beef and Bacon Hash

Yield: 4 servings

Prep Time: 30 min

Cook Time: 6 hours

Ingredients

- 6 cups beef broth

- 2 teaspoons onion powder

- 1 teaspoon celery salt

- 3 Tablespoons minced onions

- 1 teaspoon salt

- ½ teaspoon black pepper

- 1 (2-pound) rump roast

- 4 Idaho potatoes, peeled and halved

- 2 large carrots, peeled and halved

-

1 large onion, peeled and medium diced

-

4 slices bacon

-

8 eggs, for serving (optional)

Directions:

1.

Add the beef broth to the crock pot (See Kelly's Notes), and then stir in the onion powder, celery salt, minced onions, salt and pepper.

2.

Add the roast, potatoes and carrots to the crock pot and set it to LOW. Allow the roast and vegetables to cook in the crock pot for 6 hours, or until tender.

3.

Remove the cooked roast and vegetables from the crock pot and dice everything into bite-sized pieces. Combine the mixture with the diced white onion.

4.

Saute the bacon in a large skillet, reserving the drippings. Set the cooked bacon aside.

5.

Add the hash mixture to the skillet containing the bacon grease and and fry the hash until crispy, about 10 minutes. Chop up the bacon and add it to the skillet, tossing to combine.

6.

If desired, fry 2 eggs per person in a separate pan and serve the hash topped with the fried eggs.

Spaghetti Sauce

Ingredients

- 2 lb bulk Italian pork sausage or ground beef

- 2 large onions, chopped (2 cups)

- 2 cups sliced fresh mushrooms (6 oz)

- 3 cloves garlic, finely chopped

- 1 can (28 oz) Muir Glen® organic diced tomatoes, undrained

- 2 cans (15 oz each) tomato sauce

- 1 can (6 oz) tomato paste

- 1 tablespoon dried basil leaves

- 1 teaspoon dried oregano leaves

- 1 tablespoon sugar

- 1/2 teaspoon salt

- 1/2 teaspoon pepper

◌
1/2 teaspoon crushed red pepper flakes

Directions:

1.

Spray 5-quart slow cooker with cooking spray. In 12-inch skillet, cook sausage, onions, mushrooms and garlic over medium heat about 10 minutes, stirring occasionally, until sausage is no longer pink; drain.

2.

Spoon sausage mixture into cooker. Stir in remaining ingredients. Cover; cook on Low heat setting 8 to 9 hours.

Spicy Hamburger Goulash

Ingredients

- 1 pound ground beef

- 4 cans (14.5 ounces) diced tomatoes

- 1 can (4 ounces) diced green chilies

- 1 ½ cups cooked pinto beans

- 1 ½ cups cooked navy beans

- ½ cup chopped onion

- ½ cup chopped green pepper

- 2 tablespoons chili powder 1 teaspoon cumin

- 1 tablespoon Worcestershire sauce

- 2 teaspoons beef bouillon granules

- 1 teaspoon dried basil

⟩

¼ teaspoon white pepper

⟩

2 cups broken noodles

Directions:

1.

Brown your hamburger in a skillet. Transfer to a greased crock.

2.

Stir in tomatoes, chilies, beans, onion, green pepper, chili powder, cumin, Worcestershire, beef bouillon, basil, and white pepper.

3.

Cover and cook on low for five hours.

4.

Stir in broken up noodles.

5.

Return lid and cook an additional 30 minutes or until noodles are tender.

Taco Meat

Ingredients

☐
½ pound ground hamburger, browned

☐
2 cups frozen corn

☐
½ cup chopped onion

☐
1 can (14.5 ounces) diced tomatoes with green chilies

☐
1 can (8 ounces) tomato sauce

☐
1 teaspoon cumin

☐
1 teaspoon chili powder

☐
1 cup black beans, cooked

☐
Taco salad fixings: lettuce, chips, shredded cheese, sour cream

Directions

1.

Combine the meat, corn, onion, tomatoes, tomato sauce, and seasonings in your greased crock pot. Stir well.

2.

Cover and cook on low for 3 hours.

3.

Add black beans and stir.

4.

Turn off crock pot and let mixture sit to warm beans.

5.

Serve meat on top of a taco salad.

Sweet 'n Sour Pork

Ingredients

-
4 Whole yellow onions, halved and sliced

-
4-6 cloves of garlic, crushed and divided

-
1 bay leaf

-
1 Teaspoon black pepper

-
3 Pound boneless pork shoulder or butt, cut into 1 inch cubes

-
1/2 Cup apple cider vinegar

-
1/2 Cup lite soy sauce

-
1 Tablespoon sugar or sugar substitute

Directions

1.

Spread half of the onions in bottom of slow cooker. Add 2 garlic cloves, the bay leaf and pepper.

2.

Arrange pork in a single layer on top of onions. Top with remaining onions and garlic.

3.

Drizzle vinegar and soy cause over all and sprinkle with sugar.

4.

Cover and cook on HIGH for 4 hours or LOW for 8 hours.

Cranberry Apple Stuffed Pork Loin

Ingredients

3-4 pound pork loin

Apple jelly

1/4 teaspoon dried rosemary

Dried cranberries

1/2 cup apple cider or juice

2 tablespoons Worcestershire sauce

2 tablespoons apple jelly

Directions:

1.
Cut your pork loin in half lengthwise.

2.
Cover the inside with apple jelly. Sprinkle the top with rosemary.

3.
Layer dried cranberries on one side of the pork loin. Fold over and tie together.

4.

Place the loin into the crockpot with ½ a cup of apple cider or juice and a tablespoon of Worchester sauce.

5.

Combine two tablespoons of jelly and mix with one tablespoon of Worchester sauce. Cover the pork loin with your mixture.

6.

For less than 3 lbs, I cook for 1.5 hours at high per lb of meat. For a 3-4 lb pork loin, I cook on low for 6 hours or high for 5 hours. Temperature should read 145 degrees.

Easy Crock Pot Ribs

Ingredients

◻
5 pounds ribs, any style

◻
2 teaspoons garlic powder

◻
2 teaspoons onion powder

◻
2 teaspoons chili powder

◻
1 teaspoon salt

◻
6 tablespoons sucanat (or brown sugar)

◻
5 tablespoons ketchup

◻
¼ cup water

◻
½ teaspoon Worcestershire sauce

◻
½ teaspoon dry mustard

◻
½ teaspoon paprika

◻
1 teaspoon salt

⬜

¼ teaspoon pepper

⬜

4 tablespoons cornstarch

⬜

4 tablespoons water

Directions:

1.

Combine garlic powder, onion powder, chili powder, and 1 teaspoon salt. Rub into meat.

2.

Lay ribs in the bottom of a 5-6 quart greased crock pot. Layer if necessary.

3.

Combine sucanat, ketchup, water, Worcestershire, mustard, paprika, salt, and pepper. Whisk to combine.

4.

Pour over meat.

5.

Cover and cook on low for 8 hours – until meat has a temperature of 170 degrees.

6.

Remove meat from crock and keep warm.

7.

Skim grease from sauce if desired (I don't).

8.

Combine cornstarch and water. Stir into juices.

9.

Cover and cook on HIGH for 30 minutes or until thickened. Serve sauce over meat.

Pasta with Pork Ragu

Ingredients

- 1 carrot, large, chopped

- 1 onion, medium, chopped

- 1 garlic clove, chopped

- 2 T. tomato paste

- 2 tsp. thyme, dried

- 1 tsp. oregano, dried

- Kosher salt and black pepper

- 14.5 oz. tomatoes, diced, canned

- 1 1/2 lb. pork, boneless, shoulder or butt, trimmed and cut in half

- 3/4 lb. fettuccini

- Grated Parmesan, for serving

Directions:

1.

In a 4-6 quart slow cooker, combine the carrot, onion, garlic, tomato paste, thyme, oregano, 3/4 tsp. salt, and 1/4 tsp. pepper.

2.

Add the tomatoes (and the juices); add the pork and turn to coat.

3.

Cover. Cook on Low for 7-8 hours or on High for 5-6 hours, or until the pork is very tender.

4.

Twenty minutes before serving, cook the fettuccine according to the directions on the package, drain and return to the pot.

5.

Meanwhile, using 2 forks, shred the pork and mix it into the cooking liquid.

6.

Toss the pasta with the Ragu and sprinkle with Parmesan.

Parmesan Honey Pork Roast

Ingredients

- 2 - 3 lbs. pork roast, boneless

- 2/3 c. Parmesan cheese, grated

- 1/2 c. honey

- 3 T. soy sauce

- 2 T. basil, dried

- 2 T. garlic, minced

- 2 T. olive oil

- 1/2 tsp. salt

- Gravy:

- 2 T. cornstarch

- 1/4 c. water, cold

Directions:

1.

Spray slow cooker with non-stick cooking spray.

2.

Place roast in slow cooker.

3.

In a bowl, combine cheese, honey, soy sauce, basil, garlic, oil and salt; pour over pork.

4.

Cover. Cook on Low for 6-7 hours or until a meat thermometer reads 160°.

5.

Remove pork to a serving platter; keep warm.

6.

Skim fat from cooking juices; transfer to a small saucepan. Bring liquid to a boil.

7.

Combine cornstarch and water until smooth.

8.

Gradually stir into pan. Bring to a boil; cook and stir for 2 minutes or until thickened.

Mexican Pork Roast

Ingredients

?
1 2-lb. pork roast

?
1 small onion, peeled, ends removed, sliced

?
2 cloves garlic, minced or grated

?
1 c. water

?
1 tbsp. cumin

?
1 tbsp. chili powder

?
¼ tsp. black pepper

?
1 tsp. sea salt

?
1 cup dry pinto or black beans, soaked overnight

Directions

1.

Add everything to the crockpot and cook 3 – 4 hours on high, or 6 – 8 hours on low.

2.

Before serving, use two forks to pull the meat apart.

3.

You can use a slotted spoon to remove the beans from the crockpot first (if, for example, you have some family members who don't care for them), or you can mix it all together.

4.

 Serve over lettuce, or put in tortillas.

5.

Makes 6 – 8 servings.

Pork Roast with Apples & Sweet Potatoes

Ingredients

- lb pork roast

- 2 fuji apples, cored and chopped

- medium sweet potato, chopped in large pieces

- medium onion, chopped in large pieces

- tbsp minced garlic

- cup apple juice (or white grape juice or water)

- tsp sea salt

- ½ tsp black pepper

- ½ tsp ground cinnamon

- ½ tsp dried basil

- ½ tsp dried rosemary

-

½ tsp dried marjoram

-

¼ - ½ tsp crushed red pepper flakes (to taste)

Directions:

1.

Spray the bottom and sides of a 4.5 quart slow cooker.

2.

Place half of the apple, sweet potato, and onion chunks in the bottom of the slow cooker. Place the roast on top, followed by the juice.

3.

Sprinkle the herbs and spices over the roast, followed by the remaining chunks of apple, sweet potato and onion. Cover and cook on low for 6-8 hours or high for 3.5 – 4.5 hours.

4.

Once finished, remove and slice the pork roast. Scoop the apple, sweet potato, and onion chunks into a bowl and mash with a potato masher.

5.

Serves 4

Smothered Chops with Onions and Bacon

Ingredients:

- 4 ounces bacon (about 4 slices), chopped

- 3 onions, halved and sliced ½ inch thick

- 4 teaspoons brown sugar

- 3 garlic cloves, minced

- tablespoon minced fresh thyme or 1 teaspoon dried

- ⅓ cup all-purpose flour

- cup low-sodium chicken broth

- ¼ cup soy sauce

- bay leaves

- 6 7-ounce bone-in blade-cut pork chops, about ¾ inch thick, sides slit to prevent curling

- Salt and pepper

-

tablespoon cider vinegar

-

tablespoon minced fresh parsley

Directions:

1.
Cook bacon in 12-inch skillet over medium heat until crisp, 5 to 7 minutes; transfer to slow cooker. Pour off all but 2 tablespoons bacon fat left in skillet.

2.
Add onions, 1 teaspoon sugar, garlic, and thyme to fat in skillet and cook over medium-high heat until onions are softened and well browned, about 10 minutes. Stir in flour and cook for 1 minute. Slowly whisk in broth, scraping up any browned bits and smoothing out and lumps; transfer to slow cooker.

3.
Stir remaining tablespoon sugar, soy sauce, and bay leaves into slow cooker. Season pork chops with salt and pepper and nestle into slow cooker. Cover and cook until pork is tender, 6 to 8 hours on low or 3 to 5 hours on high.

4.
Transfer pork chops to serving platter, tent loosely with aluminum foil, and let rest for 10 minutes.

5.

Let braising liquid settle for 5 minutes, then remove fat from surface using large spoon.

6.

Discard bay leaves. Stir in vinegar and parsley and season with salt and pepper to taste. Spoon 1 cup sauce over chops and serve with remaining sauce.

Sweet Balsamic Glazed Pork Loin

YIELD: SERVES 6-8

Ingredients

Pork:

- 2 pound boneless pork loin roast, trimmed of large fat pockets

- 1 teaspoon ground sage

- 1/2 teaspoon salt

- 1/2 teaspoon pepper

- 1 clove garlic, finely minced or crushed

- 1/2 cup water

Glaze:

- 1/2 cup brown sugar, light or dark

- 1 tablespoon cornstarch

- 1/4 cup balsamic vinegar

-

1/2 cup water

-

2 tablespoons soy sauce

Directions:

1.

In a small bowl, combine the sage, salt, pepper and garlic.

2.

Rub the spices all over the roast.

3.

Place the pork roast in the slow cooker and pour in the 1/2 cup water. Cover and cook on low for 6-8 hours.

4.

Near the end of the cooking time for the roast, combine the ingredients for the glaze in a small saucepan and bring the mixture to a boil, then reduce and let the mixture simmer, stirring occasionally, until it thickens.

5.

Remove the pork from the slow cooker, shred and place on a platter or plate. Drizzle the glaze over the pork and serve.

Salt Crusted Pork Roast

Ingredients

- 2-3 pound Pork Sirloin Roast

Seasoning Blend

- 1 Tablespoon salt

- 1 Tablespoon black pepper

- 1 teaspoon garlic powder

- 1 teaspoon paprika

- 1 teaspoon dry sweet basil

- 1 teaspoon ground sage

Instructions

1.

Mix the seasoning blend together in a small bowl

2.

Pat dry the roast and rub seasoning blend into meat, coating well

3.

Brown the roast on the stove top over medium heat, 2-3 minutes on all sides until you get a nice carmelization

4.

Cook in a slow cooker for 8 hours on the keep warm setting until internal temperature is 145 F

5.

Remove from cooker and allow to rest for 5-10 minutes before slicing

Ham, Green Beans, & Potatoes

Ingredients

SERVINGS 6-8

- 1smoked pork hock

- 1(15 ounce) jarwhole white pearl onions

- 1(16 ounce) packagecooked diced ham (or leftover sliced ham)

- 1(16 ounce) bag frozen French-cut green beans (or regular cut, or canned)

- 4baking potatoes, diced (or red potatoes, halved)

Directions:

1.
Combine all ingredients in crock pot. (There's no need to defrost any ingredients that have been frozen.).

2.
Cook on low for 6 hours.

BACON & CHEESE QUICHE

Ingredients

- 1 tablespoon butter

- 10 eggs, beaten

- 1 cup light cream or half & half

- 8 ounces shredded cheddar cheese

- ½ teaspoon black pepper

- 10 pieces cooked bacon, chopped

- ½ cup chopped spinach

Directions:

1.

Grease the slow cooker crock with the butter (leave excess in the crock); set aside.

2.

In a large mixing bowl, combine the eggs, cream, cheese, spinach and pepper, then add to the slow cooker.

3.

Sprinkle the cooked bacon over the top of the mixture.

4.

Cover and cook on LOW for 4 hours.

5.

Keep an eye on it. Do not overcook or the quiche will be dry.

Bacon-Wrapped Pork Loin Roast

Ingredients

- 1 1/2 to 2 lb pork loin roast

- 6 to 8 slice bacon, uncooked

- salt and pepper to taste

Directions:

1.
Wash pork roast and pat dry.

2.
Add salt and pepper to taste.

3.
Wrap pork roast in uncooked bacon slices, securing underneath the roast.

4.
Cook in crockpot on low heat for about 5 to 6 hours or until bacon is cooked and roast is tender.

5.
Transfer to serving platter.

6.
Pour broth into a sauce pan and bring to a boil.

7.

Thicken using about 2 teaspoons of cornstarch mixed with enough milk to make a pourable paste. Add cornstarch mixture to broth a little at a time, whisking constantly .

SWEET & SPICY PORK PICADILLO

Ingredients

- 1 TBSP olive oil

- 1 Diced Yellow Onion

- 2 cloves minced garlic

- 1 lb boneless pork country style ribs cut into 1 inch cubes

- 1 can (14 oz) diced tomatoes undrained

- 3 tbsp cider vinegar

- 2 chipotle peppers in adobe sauce chopped (optional)

- ½ cup raisins chopped

- ½ tsp cumin

- ½ tsp ground cinnamon

- salt and pepper to taste

Directions:

1.

Heat oil in skilled over medium low heat until hot. Cook and Stir onion and garlic until translucent about 4 minutes.

2.

Add pork to skillet an brown. Transfer to crockpot

3.

Combine Tomatoes with juice, vinegar, chipotles, raisins, cumin & cinnamon in medium bowl. Pour over pork.

4.

Cover and cook on low 5 hours or high 3 hours. or until pork is fork tender.

5.

Shred pork using 2 forks. Cook 30 minutes longer. Adjust seasonings before serving with rice.

Lamb Curry

Ingredients

▢
1 ½ pound lamb (leave in large pieces, so it will be easier to remove) chicken and beef are also a good substitute

▢
1 large onion, diced

▢
2 garlic cloves, minced

▢
3 tablespoons curry powder (ours has ground coriander, turmeric, cumin, fenugreek, yellow mustard, white pepper, ginger, cinnamon, chili powder, cloves, cardamom, fennel)

▢
1 teaspoon garam masala

▢
Salt and pepper

▢
½ cup sour cream, yogurt or buttermilk

Directions:

1.
Put the onions and garlic in the crock pot and stir in the curry powder and garam masala.

2.

Add the meat and sprinkle with a little more curry powder and some salt and pepper.

3.

Cook on high 1 hour and then low 5 hours.

4.

Carefully remove the meat and then puree the onions, garlic and meat juices with an immersion blender.

5.

Shred the meat (removing any bones!) and return it to the crockpot.

6.

Stir in the sour cream (or yogurt or buttermilk) and add more curry powder, salt or pepper, as needed.

7.

Serve over rice or couscous.

Seafood Paella

Ingredients:

- 3/4 c. chopped sweet peppers

- 1/2 c. chopped onion

- 2 cloves garlic, minced

- 2 1/2 cups chicken broth

- 1 c. uncooked brown rice

- 1/2 tsp. dried thyme

- 1/4 tsp. crushed red pepper

- 1/4 tsp. ground tumeric

- 12 oz. fresh or frozen shrimp, thawed, peeled and halved

- 6 oz. canned or pouched wild-caught pink salmon, flaked

- 1 c. frozen peas

Method:

1.

Grease crock pot and add all veggies except peas. In a medium sauce pan, combine chicken broth, rice and spices.

2.

Heat until boiling, then pour over veggies in the crock pot. Cover and cook on low for 4 hours.

3.

After about 3 hours, add the shrimp, salmon and peas. Once done, let stand for about 10 minutes before serving.

4.

Serves 6.

Beans and Rice

❓
3 cups cooked beans, total

❓
1 cup brown rice

❓
1 can of diced tomatoes or 1 ½ cups fresh diced tomatoes

❓
1 tablespoon butter, melted

❓
Salt to taste

❓
1 teaspoon cumin

❓
½ teaspoon garlic powder

❓
2 cups water

❓
Diced green chilies, if desired

❓
Hot sauce or cayenne pepper, if desired

Directions:

1.
Combine rice and butter in the crock pot.

2.

Rinse and drain beans.

3.

Put remaining ingredients and beans into crock. Stir well.

4.

Cover and cook on high for 2-3 hours. Begin checking at 2 to 2 ½ hours to see if your rice is done.

Garlic Basil Pasta Sauce

Ingredients

- 28 oz. jar/can whole peeled tomatoes (3 Tbsp. extra virgin olive oil

- tsp. chopped garlic

- tsp. chopped basil

- Sea salt and pepper to taste

- If you are using fresh garlic, heat a bit of the oil and all of the garlic in a sauce pan on the stove until the garlic turns golden. Then, add garlic to the crock pot.

Directions:

1.
Add oil to the crock pot.

2.
Add tomatoes to the crock pot.

3.
Add basil to the crock pot.

4.
Add salt to the crock pot.

5.

Add pepper to the crock pot.

6.

Stir things around a bit.

7.

Let sauce cook for 4 hours on high.

OVERNIGHT CHICKEN STOCK

Ingredients

- Leftover chicken bones or carcass roughly equivalent to one small or medium sized chicken

- onion, peeled and loosely chopped

- rib of celery, roughly chopped

- carrot, roughly chopped (no need to peel)

- bay leaf

- sprig fresh parsley

- sprig fresh thyme

- Salt, to taste

Directions:

1.
After removing all edible meat from the chicken put/leave the bones, skin, cooking juices, etc. in the crock pot.

2.

Add the onion, celery, carrot and spices on top of the bones and fill the crock pot almost to the top with tap water (leaving about ½" at the top).

3.

Turn the slow cooker onto "low" after dinner and cook all night long or alternatively you could start it in the morning and cook on "low" for 8 – 10 hours during the day.

4.

After the stock is done cooking turn off the heat and, using a soup ladle, pass the stock through a fine sieve to remove all herbs/bones/etc.

5.

Either refrigerate or freeze the stock for future use. Enjoy!

Garden Marinara Sauce

Ingredients

- ½ lb of fresh garden tomatoes, peeled and roughly chopped (or 2 – 28-oz. cans.

- 2 – 5 cloves of garlic, peeled and roughly chopped

- 1 onion, peeled and roughly chopped

- About 2 cups of chopped eggplant 1 ½ Tablespoons of brown sugar/sucanat

- 1 ½ Tablespoons of Italian Seasoning

- 2 bay leaves

- A few teaspoons of finely chopped fresh herbs (I used rosemary, thyme, basil, & tarragon)

- 1 Tablespoon of Pesto (I used my homemade pesto, but store-bought is ok too)

- 1 teaspoon salt (add more or less to taste)

- Freshly ground pepper, to taste

Directions:

1. Toss everything in the crockpot except for the salt and pepper.
2. You don't have to worry about chopping things too finely because we're going to blend this all up at the end.
3. Cover and cook on low heat for at least 8 hours.
4. Remove the bay leaves and, using an immersion or regular blender, blend up the sauce, pulsing lightly for chunky sauce or blend it fine if you like a smoother sauce.
5. Add salt and pepper to taste.

Hoppin' John

Ingredients

⬚
45 ounces of cooked beans (or three cans) rinsed and drained

⬚
1 onion, chopped

⬚
1 green pepper, chopped

⬚
½ TBS granulated garlic

⬚
1 tsp cayenne pepper•

⬚
4 cups vegetable broth (I used my own recipe for vegetable broth powderand mixed it up myself.)

⬚
1 tsp salt

⬚
1 tsp pepper

⬚
1 tsp basil

⬚
1 tsp thyme

⬚
2 big splashes of hot sauce

Directions:

1.

Let this cook for 3-4 hours.

2.

Serve it alone, over rice, or with cornbread.

3.

This recipe should serve about six.

Venison Roast

Ingredients

⬚
1 venison roast (fresh or frozen)

⬚
2 cups water or stock (venison stock, beef stock, chicken stock – whatever ya got!)

⬚
1 medium onion diced or 3 Tbsp dry onion

⬚
2 garlic cloves, diced or 2 tsp garlic powder

⬚
Salt and Pepper to taste (do use some salt even if it is just a pinch)

⬚
3 Tbsp butter

⬚
1 tsp paprika

⬚
1 tsp thyme

⬚
1 tsp rosemary

⬚
5-10 potatoes (depending on size) quartered

⬚
1 cup diced/chopped carrots

Directions:

1.

Place roast in crock pot and add water or stock.

2.

Add butter by placing it on top of roast.

3.

Add remaining spices and onion.

4.

Potatoes and carrots may be added at this time if you're headed out for the day or you can add them about two hours prior to serving time.

5.

Cook on low 10 hours or high 6 hours.

Pizza Sauce

- 4, 6oz cans tomato paste (organic preferred)

- 1, 15oz can tomato sauce (organic preferred)

- 1 cup water

- 1 teaspoon garlic powder

- 2 tablespoons Italian seasoning

- 1 teaspoon salt

- ½ teaspoon pepper

- 3 tablespoons olive oil

- 1 tablespoon honey

- 4 tablespoons Parmesan cheese

Directions:

1.

Combine all ingredients except cheese in crock pot.

2.

Cover and cook on low for 4 hours.

3.

Stir every 30 minutes to 1 hour so it won't stick.

4.

After four hours, stir in cheese.

5.

Cool to room temperature and package for freezing or use in 1-2 days.

Slow Cooker Sweet Potatoes

Ingredients

- 5-7 sweet potatoes, peeled and cut into small cubes {can sub yams instead}

o
cup applesauce

- 1/3 cup packed brown sugar

o
tablespoons butter, melted

o
1/2 teaspoon cinnamon

- 1/2 cup toasted pecans

Directions

1.
In a small mixing bowl, stir applesauce, brown sugar, butter and cinnamon together. Lay sweet potatoes in the bottom of a slow cooker.

2.
Pour applesauce mixture over potatoes.

3.
Cover and cook on low until potatoes are tender, about 6-8 hours.

4.

Use an immersion blender or potato masher until nice and smooth.

5.

Sprinkle with nuts and serve.

Pumpkin and Coconut Black Beans and Rice

Prep time: 10 mins

Cook time: 8 hours

Total time: 8 hours 10 mins

Serves: a crowd

Ingredients

- 1 green pepper, chopped (Optional. I've done it both ways, and either way is great.)

- 1 large yellow onion, chopped

- 2 cloves garlic, minced

- 1 lb. black beans, rinsed

- 1 or 2 cups pumpkin puree (How much do you like pumpkin?)

- 4 tablespoons tomato paste

- 1 tablespoon curry powder

- 1 teaspoon cayenne pepper (more if you don't have little ones)

- 1 teaspoon cumin

- 1 bay leaf

- 1 can coconut milk

- 1 Tablespoon kosher salt

- 3 cups chicken stock

- 3 cups water or 6 cups if you don't have stock

- Cilantro

- Plain yogurt

Instructions

1.
Saute green pepper and onion for 5 minutes.

2.
Add garlic and saute for another minute.

3.
Add sauteed vegetables and all other ingredients except cilantro and yogurt to slow-cooker

4.

Set the slow-cooker on high and let it go about 8 hours.

5.

Check water level from time to time, adding more if necessary to prevent burning.

6.

Garnish with cilantro and a dollop of plain yogurt.

7.

Southwestern Bean Medley

- 14 ounces vegetable broth

- Tbsp chili powder

- tsp ground cumin

- can black beans

- can chickpeas

- can white kidney beans (cannellini)

- 1/2 C dried lentils

- C diced tomatoes with green chilies

Directions:

1.
Copped fresh cilantro leaves

2.
Mix all ingredients except tomatoes and cilantro in 3 1/2 quart slow cooker (or whatever size you happen to have). Cover and cook on low 6 to 7 hours. Add tomatoes. Cover and cook for 1 hour. Sprinkle with cilantro.

Potato Breakfast

- 2 large baking potatoes, sliced thick

- 1 medium onion, sliced

- 1 cup shredded cheese

- ½ cup chopped peppers

- 1 tablespoon + butter

- Meat

Directions

1.
Layer the potatoes, onion, cheese, meat, and peppers in a greased crock pot.

2.
Sprinkle top with salt and pepper.

3.
Dot butter over top of mixture.

4.
Cover and cook on low for 6-8 hours, depending on thickness of the potatoes.

Macaroni and Cheese

- 1/2 pound uncooked elbow macaroni (regular, gluten free, spelt, you name it on the variety of noodle)

- 3 cups shredded Cheddar cheese, divided

- 3 cups whole milk (I use goat milk)

- 2 eggs

- ½-1 teaspoon garlic salt

- 1/2 teaspoon ground black pepper

- 1/2 teaspoon mustard powder

Directions:

1.
Mix all ingredients except 1/2 cup cheese in a slow cooker, then sprinkle the remaining cheese on top.

2.
Cover and cook on low for 5 hours. Enjoy!